Feed Thy Gut 2

Go Heal Yourself!

David Podlipny

ISBN-13: 979-8-5865-4973-0

This book has been written purely for informational and entertainment purposes, and is not a substitute for professional medical care. The author is not responsible for any specific health or allergy needs that may require medical supervision and is not liable for any loss, injury, damage or negative consequences from any treatment, action, application or preparation, to any person reading or following the information in this book. References and links are provided for informational purposes only and do not constitute endorsement of any websites or other sources, and readers should be aware that the websites listed in this book may change. The author assumes no responsibility for errors or changes that occur after publication with regards to the internet addresses provided.

Contents

When health is absent, wisdom cannot reveal itself, art cannot manifest, strength cannot fight, wealth becomes useless, and intelligence cannot be applied.

Herophilus (Greek physician, c. 335–c. 280 BC)

Back at It Again

Every now and then I come across a lifestyle piece, be it in a magazine, on TV, or online, saying something along the lines of; despite being afflicted with a severe disease like multiple sclerosis (MS), thanks to the many wonders of modern medicine, person A can now live a productive, active, and happy life. Behold person A smiling at you from a children's swing. Then they outline the list of medications person A is taking, and their history of disabilities. But don't despair; they try to live each day with as much laughter as possible, and they trust their doctors, the entire medical establishment; person A wants to thank them from the bottom of their heart, and person A's children wants to thank them as well.

(I sincerely hope all that daily laughter is the result of some quality, home-grown weed.)

All I can think of, all my mind is flooded with after absorbing these kinds of things, is *goddammit, this is all so fucking unnecessary*... (Yes, there will be the occasional curse word here and there. Or, actually, lots of them. Go ahead; dump buckets of smelling salts around you to quickly get back to your feet...

and hopefully consciousness *before* defying gravity.)

Why I think it's so goddamn unnecessary?

Because I'm a snob.

I actually am. Have become. (Always was?)

Is there anything wrong with person A, or their account? No.

(Because person A is imaginary?) No!

I have very little to spare in terms of sympathy for people talking (complaining!) about their MS; especially those on medications, taking the traditional path. Any autoimmune disease for that matter.

(Because I'm jealous? Could be. Because they've accepted it, the medicine is working, and they're being looked after? Maybe the last one, but the rest... nah-uh.)

My default response to sick people expressing a complaint nowadays is: stop whining. Which is a rather dangerous stance, since I can easily dismiss genuine complaints...

But if I didn't have MS myself, I couldn't complain about other people that have it?

Fuck you!

(How brave of me to go out on a limb like that! A limb that fell to the ground decades ago...)

I look down on everyone with multiple sclerosis that hasn't gone full hippie weirdo simply because my head is ballooning with hot air. In a wheelchair?

Loser! Hunched over a cane? Weakling! Complain about numbness? Ignoramus! You could all live a better life. Healthier, happier. With less disability, pain, fatigue, brain fog, rage, and overall misery. What about the holy grail—productivity? Ah... I hate that word. But what the hell; since I'm feeling megalomaniacal (or is it magnanimous?) you can all be extra productive too! And for all of you that weren't, welcome up to ground level; to humanity.

Yes, I actually think all of that. *Better* lives... who the hell does this jerk think he is?

Messiah!

That's who.

Messiah!

Sorry. It's just fun to scream. Try it.

Messiah!

I don't do this every time... the disparaging asshole thing. Just whenever I can't suppress it, or hide it somehow. Gloss it over with fake altruism.

Mess... no. No.

We're off to a great start! I hate myself already. Two jars of peanut butter will suffocate my sorrows. If I can get it down, and won't choke on it first.

Win win?

I could blame the progress I've made over the years for my lack of sympathy toward suffering, but that's a pretty ass-backwards way of approaching it. Moreover since I know that it's all my own doing. At times it's like I'm convinced I don't suffer anymore; I've successfully abolished it, just by adjusting my aim, by going down this "divine" road... I've made myself *in*human in pursuit of this luminous thing. Great. I'm blind instead.

Besides, who am I to tell anyone what to do? I hate it when people tell me what to do. More so when they're doing it in a disparaging way, treating me like I've just hit my head and the resulting bump is a concave one. All right, I don't hate it; I dislike it. Then when I think about it, I actually turn to loathing; loathing myself for being such a hardheaded oaf. Be more open; accepting.

Is that what you want to hear? My road to redemption? My enlightenment?

I'm such a great liar.

This self-deprecating spiel intended to sneakily gain favor is getting tedious...

And if I was a doctor? A doctor with good intentions? (Now now, that's no way to behave.) Would that change anything? Would that give me the stamp of approval to do this?

As long as you're productive and active, *everything* will be all right...

Can you please just get on with the book? Nobody wants to hear these unhinged ramblings, this cerebral diarrhea... and the spoiled cherry on top where you undercut everything you say.

(A performative lunacy?)

Shush. Proceed we shall!

It's not like my own life is the epitome of virtue, health, and happiness. The number of times I've sabotaged things for myself are uncountable. It scares me just to ponder it. Some are hilarious and idiotic. But most of them are just plain ugly; chronic exercises in feelings of unworthiness. Inferiority circle jerks. If there's one thing I can take to the bank, it's that no matter what, no matter how great of a progress I've made, how glorious the present moment is, I'm going to find a way to sabotage it.

One way or another, I always find a way.

Always...

Just stop doing it, silly. You deserve to be happy!

Deserve? Do I, really? On what grounds? Just by breathing, by being alive?

No. Just accepting that at face value could break my spirits. Luckily I'm all stocked up.

Mamajuana. Look it up.

And that's just talking about the health piece of the pie, the whole quest to rid myself of disease and various ailments and complaints; multiple sclerosis, acne, and depression. Among many things...

Maybe that's the problem; the binary, black or white sort of thinking that's so ingrained in me. Either fix me up for good, or just leave me to die. Well, not that dramatic maybe... but definitely closer to an extremist view than a lax one. You're never going to be healthy, so why even bother?

Yes... *darkness*.

Like I even know what good health entails. The real meaning of true wealth? The ability to roundhouse kick adversity in the face?

Good by what standards?

It changes from day to day; from moment to moment. I guess it's to a large part subjective. Does that mean I'm chasing a specter? Not necessarily. I do believe there is an overarching—or underlying—structure to strive for, an amorphous stability of sorts, a velvety feeling of trust, which necessarily doesn't have a name or a face, but when you've reached it, you'll know. And when you're not there, you know too. Perhaps the latter is much more concrete than anything else.

Unleash the W's! Wishy-washy, woo-woo malarkey.

Nowadays, there is so much to choose from, so much information available on health that it's discombobulating.

(Bobulate, Disco M. Bobulate. *That* would be my secret-agent name.)

Which is a good thing; it gives everyone the chance to take their health into their own hands. But besides being a daunting task, it can also be a great risk. Though one doesn't have to go all in; you're not simply left to the mercy of your doctor anymore. Autonomy of virtually every level is now present. Treatment can be endlessly tailored.

The problem is how to sort through all of it; it's all too easy to get lost in the health jungle, and go bankrupt in the process. But more and more evidence is building up in favor of food and various lifestyle changes as excellent complements or even replacing conventional medicines. For many chronic conditions, the key to getting well is no longer about getting the right lineup of drugs.

And as long as there's an open discussion, a transparent debate happening, we'll cope, and hopefully, advance along the way.

But unfortunately, information alone is not enough to change behavior. Life would be so much easier if it were... even if it's scientifically vetted, and thousands of people swear by it. Sure, it might lend it some, or even a lot of credibility, but ultimately the decision has to come from within oneself. Any other way is doomed to fail.

Is it really unfortunate, that information isn't enough to change behavior? What if the experts are in fact charlatans? The people who swear by it have all been paid off? Or the gatekeepers only allow what they deem appropriate through the gates, acting on an agenda that goes completely contrary to the public good?

What's worse is that two of the perhaps biggest contributors, the sectors with the most clout, have been virtually blind to the many ways they're interconnected: the food industry doesn't factor in the health aspect, and the medical industry doesn't factor in the food aspect. But maybe that's slowly changing, very slowly. It's hard to tell for sure, whether it's just a cosmetic change, or something is actually happening deeper down. I'm hopeful. Baby steps are better than Brontosaurus steps.

In all likelihood, I would never have started this whole health quest unless I got MS. I was doing all kinds of stuff to combat the acne, but that was more from the medical side; antibiotics, ointments and creams and whatnot. I didn't even think you could do anything much about depression except popping pills with evocative names. I guess I didn't delve much into any of it when I was younger... just give me whatever fixes it.

Why would I change anything had I not been diagnosed with MS? Change life *so* drastically? I'm basically a self-made pariah when it comes to all matters concerning food; anything that I haven't prepared myself or seen the ingredients beforehand, is no bueno. No bu-ey-no. But then I've also taken a rather extreme stance...

(You're using highly-processed canola oil? What the fuck is wrong with you? Yes, it might kill me if I eat it just once! You're a terrible cook...)

Only once I hit a new low did I feel the need to change anything: when my body got a life of its own, my limbs a mind of their own, all alien to me; or simply just stopped altogether—that freaked me out. Freaked me out enough to go searching for an alternative. There really wasn't anywhere else to go. All right, there was, and yes, suicide was in the picture too. At times suicide took up the entire picture, while I tried to get its heavy feet off my chest. But the allure of a "normal", disease-free life was too big. Too enchanting. I had seen what such a life could look like. I had seen it in movies. I had dreams! Sexy dreams...

You should've been proactive, silly! Don't wait until the illness has taken hold of you before you start contemplating a healthier lifestyle, before you act.

That's a delusion if there ever was one...

But of course, as with everything, it's a nuanced matter. The longer you wait, the harder many diseases are to treat and the more expensive they get too. (If you have the luxury of waiting, of treatment, and of having money in the bank.)

That doesn't mean it's impossible to mitigate or reverse a disease, but if you just give someone a pill and send them off it most certainly will be.

Modern trauma care is phenomenal, but when it comes to treating chronic disease... not so much. The way we address it is to suppress the symptoms; we never get to the underlying causes. And much of it might not even need any drugs at all... or the emptying of savings accounts.

The years following the first Feed Thy Gut book have been about tweaking, perfecting; finding new ways to strengthen the body naturally; and in some cases simply dumping approaches that didn't work for me. And also about regressing a few times, though not intentionally... most of the time. In the following pages I'll outline it all. I'll dispense of the sugarcoating, or I'll try, try to make it as honest an account as I can stomach without feeling the need to move to Mars afterwards.

Which I will never do. Self-evisceration; commence! Welcome to my second, infinitely more mature whine-fest.

(And yes; I will start off each chapter with a pretentious quote. Sometimes they won't have anything to do with the subsequent chapter, sometimes they will.)

I can resist everything except temptation.

Oscar Wilde

Lady Windermere's Fan (1892)

What Didn't Work for Me

Garlic is one of the healthiest things you can eat.[1] So why shouldn't you? I sure as hell did; a few years back I remember eating three or four cloves with every meal. Even my perspiration reeked of garlic. Yum.

Granted, that was probably a bit too much, but what about regular consumption?

I didn't want to believe it—I wanted to continue eating one of the healthiest foods you can eat—but after a while it became painfully evident that my stomach didn't care much for garlic, no matter how much I tried to persuade it. Every test I performed on myself turned out the same; I felt strange, nebulously so, my stomach was bloated and a general discomfort around my stomach always persisted after I ate garlic. I tried various approaches to make sure it really was garlic; to eat it after fasting, on an empty stomach with nothing else, with varying time intervals; I tried to sneak it into various other foods as well, but nothing worked. I never really thought about garlic being problematic; it wasn't even remotely close to being on my radar, until I chanced upon an article online once, describing my symptoms down to a T. Lo and behold, when I followed the advice, removing garlic from my diet, the bloating and stomach discomfort disappeared.

Thus raw garlic became a definitive no-no for me—and its cousins onions and leeks too—although cooked or roasted worked fine for the most part, but with garlic-infused olive oil I had no stomach issues whatsoever.

The good news was that I could still get—maybe not all of the benefits, but surely some—by simply infusing oils with garlic. Some of its beneficial properties are bound to be left behind in the flesh, but a little of the good stuff is better than none.

But why is garlic so problematic for some?

Garlic is a high FODMAP food. FODMAP is an acronym for **F**ermentable **O**ligo-, **D**i-, **M**ono-saccharides **A**nd **P**olyols; short chain carbohydrates that are poorly absorbed in the small intestine—we do not possess the enzyme needed to break down the fructans in garlic into single molecules[2]. Which is not necessarily bad; they act as prebiotics (fertilizers that stimulate the growth of healthy bacteria in the gut, whereas the more commonly heard probiotics contain live organisms), and might even possess antioxidant and immunomodulatory properties[3].

Garlic is chockfull of fructo-oligosaccharides—or fructans—which belong to the oligosaccharide category, the O in FODMAP. Although garlic is a high FODMAP food, garlic-infused oil is a low FODMAP food. The reason behind that is the fructans in garlic are water soluble, and not oil soluble. Same goes for onions. Just make sure there are no itsy bitsy tiny pieces of garlic in there, if you're very sensitive to it. Strain it if you have to.

I didn't eat garlic-infused olive oil consistently. I simply made a bottle of it, and when that one was empty, I sometimes waited a week or a month before making another one. Or I made two bottles of it at once. It depended.

But I do tend to consume extra-virgin olive oil—a little bit of it poured on food—every day.

Fermented foods are supposed to be awesome too. I'm sure they are; just not for me. But that didn't stop me from consuming copious amounts of it. I have a tendency to overdo things; especially the stuff lauded as superfoods. The stuff that will get your health back.

Fermented foods, mainly sauerkraut and pickled cucumbers (salt being the only other ingredient in both), gave me symptoms pretty much identical to the ones garlic did; bloating, stomach discomfort, but also severe gas. And *smelly* gas. All day long...

Fermented white cabbage (sauerkraut) is a high FODMAP food.[4] But it could also be that the live microorganisms were wreaking havoc to my gastrointestinal highway, e.g. a histamine intolerance. Long story short, I didn't feel good eating fermented foods.

I also tried eating lots of capsaicin, mainly in the form of cayenne pepper, but also peri-peri (here it's called piri piri), to the point that it felt like fire was coming out my rear end every time I went to the toilet. Again, I'd read of the almost magical properties of capsaicin, so I went all in. Which might actually have caused damage to my gut.[5]

And now to fruit. Yes, ordinary, everyday fruit. Fruit *really* messed me up. Well, most of it did. Then again, I ate *a lot* of fruit at one point. If it's healthy, then more's got to be better, right?

(Are you starting to see a pattern here? Moderation is a word I'm only just now learning.)

Most of the time I would get incredibly tired after eating fruit, and yes, bloated too. But mostly tired; completely drained of all energy. It turns out that some people have a hard time digesting and absorbing fructose.[6]

(Are fructans, like those found in garlic for example, the same thing as fructose? A fructan is a polymer of fructose molecules, i.e. a chain of fructose molecules form a fructan. Fructans are found in certain grains and vegetables, while fructose is predominantly found in fruit, honey, molasses, and corn syrup.)

Pretty much all fruits caused problems for me, except for bananas and berries, both which are relatively low in fructose. Berries can also boast of being incredibly nutritious and provide many health benefits.[7]

I also noticed that I fare much better on less carbohydrates. But more on that later.

It took a long while for me to find these things out, or stumble across them rather. I was always so snowed in on the notion that anything deemed healthy can't possibly be bad for you, whether in small or large doses. Parents and people around me as well as society at large hail most of these things, like fruit, as unequivocally good for you. It's healthy, period. There's so much in life that passes unquestioned.

Now, coconut oil was a tricky one; it didn't really make me feel any outright discomfort, but it didn't make me feel great either. Can you guess the reason by now? I ate a lot of it. Two or three tablespoons a day. Why? Because it's so damn tasty; coupled with some coconut flakes, either roasted or raw, it becomes a fatty, velvety sort of sweetness that leaves your mouth pleasantly refreshed.

And it's healthy!

Maybe if I had Polynesian roots, I could cope with it better, maybe even thrive on it, but my European ancestors hardly saw more than a handful of coconuts in their lifetime, let alone splurged on them. Raw cabbage, here I come.

Cabbage—the coconut of Europe.

Of course, it's not always that easy to make changes, especially when it comes to food. The world today is a terribly tasty place... and when you come up against a particularly difficult opponent, things can get tricky real fast. In my case, that opponent was peanut butter. It never really finds its place in my stomach; most of the time it feels like it's trying to crawl back up. If I burp several hours later, I can still taste every ground-up peanut, like it's refusing to be digested. It just isn't worth those moments of odd pleasure it brings. But in the end I found a solution for that too, though it wasn't a pretty one: eat so much of it till you get sick of it. For me that moment occurred after I ate a whole jar; just grabbed a spoon and went to work. Genius. I know I can't stop eating it if I just will myself into it. I've willed myself to stop eating peanut butter maybe twenty times, if not more. But this worked. (For now...?)

Another way is to simply not buy it in the first place.

And finally, to the real monster: the ketogenic diet.

Blasphemy! Heretic! Burn him! (After you've doused him in duck fat.)

The ketogenic diet (or simply keto diet) swept the entire world, at least for a while. It's a high fat, very low carbohydrate diet which makes the body burn fats instead of carbohydrates, and was originally used to treat epilepsy in children. It can mitigate the symptoms of neurodegenerative diseases, diabetes, cancer, and even some autoimmune conditions.[8] A lot of the science on it seems promising, and judging by the anecdotal evidence, it is clearly helping a lot of people.

But not me. No... this one I actually regret.

Within weeks of going full keto, I noticed something was wrong, but couldn't quite put my finger on it. So I stuck with it, convinced that it was just my body adjusting to it. Over the following days and weeks, the by then dormant (what I thought was actually solved once and for all) fungal problems completely exploded. My scalp got extremely dry and crusty; my skin overall became very dry; the nail fungus returned; the athlete's foot returned; a whitish, almost cheese-like coating reappeared on my tongue; my elbows got dry and crusty; clusters of pimples appeared on strange spots like my forearms and my shins, and on my face as well.

It all came back with a vengeance. Abandoning the keto diet didn't make much of a difference either, at least not for a long while.

My left foot, or at least the sole of it, soon looked like a really disgusting, dry pastry. It was so bad that I'd repeatedly tear holes in my socks with the sharp crust on my sole, particularly around the ball of my foot, just by wearing them around the apartment. If I ever harbored or considered cultivating a foot fetish, any such fancies were now decapitated and tossed into an active volcano.

A common belief is that carbohydrates exacerbate fungal infections (or even causes them), so therefore going very low carb, or even eliminating them altogether, should solve any such problems. But the keto diet can leave some people immune deficient, especially against pathogens like fungi and parasitic worms. Carbohydrates are important for anti-fungal immunity, and going on a low carb diet can bring about some deficiencies, like Vitamin C deficiency, which also impairs anti-fungal immunity.[9]

"A lot of plant foods can really help suppress fungi in the gut and promote bacteria. So they can help give you a better gut flora and I think a lot of people who go extremely low carb can end up with a gut dysbiosis of some kind after years on these extreme low carb diets."[10]

It was such a heavy blow, so utterly demoralizing, that I thought long and hard about just giving up trying to fix my health, and eat whatever the hell I wanted to. Fuck all of this. I went all in thinking I was doing the best thing I could do to assist my body in healing, and look what happened—you're not just back where you started; you actually made it all worse.

So why didn't you just give up?

I wish I had an answer for that. I really don't know what it was; at least I can't put it into easily comprehensible words. Maybe I simply faked it. A lot of the time it felt like it was insanity more than reason that kept me going. If such a clear dichotomy even exists.

Now, it's crucial to isolate foods when testing yourself for intolerances, to ingest them separately so you know what's what. It might be incredibly tedious, but worth it in the long run. Something I learned the hard way.

Of course, you could also take the responsible, adult approach, and simply get yourself tested for various food sensitivities. I might take a food sensitivity test sometime in the future... or not. I'm not really there yet... I've come too far to turn back now: I'm going to see this thing through to the end. Pigheaded glory awaits! It would feel like giving up, at least a large part of me would feel that way, if I were to turn to a health professional at this point—surrender.

One day I had a lightbulb moment: I've never actually tested whether gluten was a problem for me, tested it under controlled circumstances. Like a *real* scientist.

Or had I? I couldn't remember. I didn't give it

much more thought and just decided to try. I fasted for 20 hours, and then had some regular, store-bought ice cream (more chocolate and caramel crunch than ice cream), along with two generic wheat cookies, also store bought. Neither of the two were caveman-friendly by any stretch of the imagination (ancestral diet, paleo-adjacent, nutrivore, omnivore, primal, hunter-gatherer, or whatever you want to call it).

The outcome was bad. *Real* bad. It started within a few hours; I felt heavy and slow, and my stomach didn't feel like my own anymore—I almost puked on several occasions. The next day, after a less than refreshing night's sleep (I did have some wild, bizarre dreams though), I woke up with a stuffed nose, and the fatigue was absolutely crushing; I had zero energy, and even though I tried to repeatedly, I just couldn't fall asleep during the day for some much-needed shuteye. In the following days I had a bunch of pimples pop up, and even an abscess on the inside of my cheek. Not until a week had passed did I feel like myself again.

I don't know how much I set myself back by pulling this stunt. Moreover, the experiment failed on so many levels: I have no idea whether it was the dairy, the wheat, or any of the twenty-plus ingredients between the ice cream and the cookies that triggered it all. So much for scientific methods.

Basically it was just an excuse—a mammoth of a pretext—for me to break the rules, taste the forbidden fruit... to LIVE! For once in my wretched life... (Cue the violins and sobbing seniors.)

Another subterfuge that only lead me deeper down the Toilet of Martyrs. A moment of weakness. And probably not the last either...

It's important to remember that this isn't a forever thing; once your gut heals, you can add stuff back. How fast and what is extremely individual. I'm reacting much better to the things I've just listed (that I want to eat)—in that there is no adverse reaction to register—and I expect that to continue, as long as I stick with it. All it takes is a great deal of patience, and trying to minimize the setbacks that will inevitable come. I've realized there is no other worthwhile mindset than to be in it for the long run. Fun.

Now, you have to be flexible (or try at least) when it comes to food, since a dogmatic approach won't get you very far; what works for some, or even the vast majority, might not work for others. Do take into account the views of experts, but first and foremost listen to your own body—personalization is key.

What I wanted to illustrate with these examples (besides being able to act foolishly, if there was still any doubt) is that some of the foods which I thought were my best friends, might in fact have hindered my improvement, or worse, caused outright harm. Always put your assumptions, your beliefs, to the test.

So that's it? Remove the foods that don't agree with you and you'll be cured of all worldly ills?

Food-related matters are only a part of the journey to a healthier body; a vital part, sure, but it's all interconnected. So what else did I do? This was merely the self-denigrating entrée, ladies and gentlemen...

Our destiny is frequently met in the very
paths we take to avoid it.

Jean de la Fontaine

Fables, Book VIII (1678–1679)

More Food-Related Harangues

I haven't had any new flare-ups since the one I had in 2013. The weakness in my entire left side (leg and arm, especially noticeable when working out), has improved to the point that I don't even feel it being there anymore. The tingling and numbness in the tips of my fingers, however, is something I still sense, though to a much lesser extent than what it used to be.

For me, changing what I ate made a world of difference. Besides multiple sclerosis, it improved (dare I say fixed?) my acne, eczema, dry skin, fungal problems, depression, insomnia, brain fog, fatigue, allergies, and—well, maybe that's enough to get the point across.

Years of doing things the conventional way, doing what the doctors told me, what was sanctioned by modern society, only pulled my body deeper into the mire, and my soul closer to the windy edge.

(Oh, the inconsistent melodrama!)

Not only is the gut-brain connection now well established[11], but more and more evidence is emerging that there is also a gut-skin connection[12].

Likely there is even more to be discovered relating to the gut and the role it plays in the rest of our bodies.

Now, I can't in good conscience claim to have deliberately sought out the uncomfortable like a respectable Stoic, or in any way opted for the dangerous, untrodden path like some golden-maned hero on an epic crusade. Most of it was just resignation from the many poor outcomes that I experienced with modern medicine—which is a luxury in itself, to be able to shun it—and a small part of it was probably out of spite too.

Toward the medical establishment which I felt had wronged me, or toward myself?

Ha… hmm.

But nonetheless, flip the script I did: I stopped taking the medication; no more needles, pills or anything, and wholeheartedly adopted a time-tested tactic: stop eating crap, or at least stop eating so much of it. Deep down we all have a general sense of what that entails; it's the details that are endlessly contested. And rightly so.

Instead of taking it easy, as everyone around me suggested—my brother being the sole exception—not exciting the immune system unnecessarily, I went in the other direction, and tried to strengthen it. Fight back. I wasn't about to become a bedridden blob.

The hygiene hypothesis[13] I believe has a lot of merit to it. Likewise with the excessive cleanliness run amok in the West today; a little dirt won't hurt. Not even a lot of it. All this; the excessive cleanliness (now that you're frail), the comfortable life (now that you're frail and sick), the victimhood (now that you're frail, sick, and deserving of pity) was a disaster for me. In the beginning I happily wallowed in it all. I was a king sitting in my very own cesspool, making titillating bubbles with a long drinking straw.

Going against all this, going my own way in a sense, brought me some much-needed agency—no, scratch that: a lot—and goddammit, did that feel good. It still fills me with crackling, sparkling energy just to know that I can change things on my own. It is equally scary for that same reason; simply because I've got to know myself better over the years—during these past ten or fifteen years especially—and I now know the person looking back at me in the mirror is an amalgamation of countless, sundry personalities. Which makes things interesting, if nothing else...

Over time it has also spilled over to other areas of my life; virtually to all of them. (There will be more on that in later chapters.) A door that, once opened, revealed not just a hidden house, but an entire hidden city.

I finally feel like I have a firm grasp of what I'm doing, where I'm heading with this; a workable blueprint that I can follow for the rest of my life, knowing that I can not only live by it, but also thrive on it. It is not a complete blueprint by any means—I'm not a concrete gazebo—but the best, up-to-date version available, and malleable enough for future adjustments. And I'm not even halfway through this journey, and already am I seeing amazing results.

Halfway through? How do I know where exactly I am on this journey, if I don't know where the finish line is? Something amorphous, like "feel better", or "get better"? When MS is dead? When I've achieved immortality?

(Cancer is a form of immortality—cells divide indefinitely. Let's aim for *that*.)

Even so, I sometimes think that if I can only get this thing to congeal, to set like cement—to be finished with it, past the finish line so to speak, whatever or wherever it is—I could finally live a normal life. But looking for something static to cling to could prove equally disastrous. Maybe impatience is a big part of that.

Maybe... how about definitely?

It took me a while, but now I'm nonetheless feeling (and seeing) great results, like I'm making actual, measurable progress. No wonder it took so long, since I had a whole grocery list of ailments when I started. I doubt I was perfectly healthy my entire life, and then suddenly one morning everything just went south—a full-systems collapse from one day to the next. More likely it was something that had built up over a long period of time. So I shouldn't expect to rid myself of something in a week or two what perhaps took months or years to entrench itself. But I can't blame my body for this; in fact, my body was trying its best to protect me, to keep me alive;[14] an immune system whose amazing efficacy the generations before me can attest to, simply by my being here. Complaining while stuffing my face with sugar-dusted macaroni and gulping down soda is all on me. (Which I did when I was younger; crap was a staple of my childhood.)

Treat your body with the respect it demands, and a lot is won. Which might be hard to do when you're younger, but as an adult the ball's in your court.

But it feels like I've gone off on a tangent here; let's get back to food.

Since my less than optimal experience with the keto diet, I haven't really tried anything else. Veganism and the carnivore diet are too extreme in my view; sure, some people seem to fare well while on them, but both lack a great deal of essential nutrients (as do vegetarians)[15, 16]. I've tried vegetarianism for a while, a long time ago, but it didn't work for me; a lot of the aforementioned problems, like bloating, fungal issues, and fatigue, quickly got out of hand. And meat, even the oft-demonized red meat[17], is an essential component of a nutritious diet[18].

And why should I try something else at this point? I'm sticking with what I'm currently doing (or trying to anyway), with what's clearly working for me.

In the end, you have to adopt a diet that you can and will stick with; until it no longer feels like a diet, like a chore—it's just the way you eat. The crap you used to eat was a diet: The Standard American Diet, aptly known as the SAD diet.

But be careful if and when you decide to ditch the SAD diet for something else (preferably food; don't go breatharian), to then view the results as evidence that the diet you're now on is a panacea. Many diets containing real food are a step up from the SAD diet, so of course things will improve... for a while; be careful of what Chris Kresser calls the honeymoon phase[19], which is to not only look at the results a month after adopting a new diet (here he is speaking specifically about veganism), but several months after, even years. You want something that will sustain you for a long time, nourish you your whole life, and not leave you deficient in vital nutrients.

Another thing is that I'm more focused on healing instead of killing now; before it was an all-out war on... on what exactly? I have no idea. The bad guys making me sick. Where's my shotgun? Whatever it was, it was going to die. The only thing that suffered in that civil war was my health. Or so I believe. It was too much, too often. There was very little balance in my aggressive method.[20]

So, what changes have I made since the last book?

I eat about a cup's worth of carbohydrates and less than a cup's worth of fruit a day, give or take; generally a little bit more carbohydrates on days with heavy workouts. It's not like I have a cup out at all times, measuring every serving, but it's a good measure to go by. That makes roughly three medium-sized potatoes a day, to give you a more palpable sense of it. The fruit is usually in the form of berries and bananas. Berries, despite being incredibly nutrient dense, are very affordable. I guess that's because they're neither sexy nor exotic, and for that I am grateful.

I eat less protein; if I was out hiking all day, climbing trees, pushing rocks, then maybe that would warrant it, but like this, staring at a screen for most of the day... not really. Extra protein is not only unnecessary; it can even be detrimental to your health.[21] And it's not like I'm going hungry, and I'm gaining muscle too[22], so there is no real need to be as protein obsessed as every other food ad wants me to be.

I eat more fat; specifically I've began eating more liver (for the most part chicken liver), as well as ghee (a class of clarified butter that originated in ancient India[23]), and I eat more vegetables as well.

When I follow this model—small to moderate

amounts of carbs and fruits, moderate amounts of protein, and lots of vegetables and fats—my stomach is happy, and my bowel movements are pleasant (no more diarrhea, cadaverous smells, stomach cramps, or bloating). I hardly ever fart anymore either, and when I do, they're not of the rotting-animal-inside-me kind.

I've got roughly the same diet as outlined in the first book, with a few important adjustments here and there:

Carbohydrates

I hardly eat legumes anymore; if I do, it's maybe once a month or even less. The bulk of my carbohydrate intake comes from regular potatoes, sweet potatoes, and white rice. The white rice I soak overnight and then rinse before cooking to significantly reduce the amount of arsenic.[24] These three (along with a few others) are what The Perfect Health Diet designates as "safe starches".[25]

Oats I try to stay away from as much as I can. Very small amounts every now and then are fine, but the hard part is not going for that extra serving, because freshly-baked oatmeal bread with a bit of ghee melting on top of it (and a pinch of salt)... holy hell that's diabolically tasty!

What's more, oatmeal bread is dangerously simple: soak oats overnight, with either something acidic in it (lemon or apple cider vinegar) or just some plain sea salt, and then plop it all out on an appropriate tray, and after an hour or so you've got yourself some very aromatic oatmeal bread.[26]

Fats

Extra virgin olive oil is a staple in my kitchen. Virgin coconut oil not so much anymore; hardly ever nowadays. I'll have a teaspoon of it every now and then, like three or four times a month maybe. But the most impactful addition has been ghee, the golden-hued, clarified butter. Ghee *is* dairy, but since the milk solids have been removed it's lactose and casein free, contains butyrate (butyric acid, a short-chain fatty acid that plays a central role in gut health) and vitamin K2; do make sure the one you get is from grass-fed cows, since it contains much higher levels of all the good stuff.[27]

You can make your own too, if you can get your hands on organic butter from cows that graze on grass. I've never tried this myself, since that kind of butter is damn-near impossible to find around here, not to mention at a reasonable price. But a quick search should give you plenty of material to browse through, if you're keen on the idea of making some homemade gold.

Vitamin K2 was also called Activator X once upon a time, coined by its discoverer Dr. Weston Price. "Vitamin K2 plays a crucial role in the development of the facial bones, and its presence in the diets of non-industrialized peoples explains the wide facial structure and freedom from dental deformities that Weston Price observed."[28] Besides dental health, it also plays a beneficial role in bone health, the health of your skin, brain[29], and kidneys[30].

"Ethnic groups that do not use butter obtain the same nutrients from things like insects, organ meats, fish eggs and the fat of marine animals, food items most of us find repulsive. For Americans—who do not eat bugs or blubber—butter is not just better, it is essential."[31]

The vitamin trio of A, D, and K can also help with dental cavities[32], and their meager presence in modern diets could be the reason behind crooked teeth[33].

I noticed a clear improvement in my dental health after implementing adequate intakes of the ADK trio—translucent tips were filled out, a dark spot on one of my molar's disappeared—as well as an improvement in the vitality of my skin. Though Superman health probably isn't attainable (as I posited in the first book), not in the foreseeable future anyhow, Superman skin however is *actually* attainable. (Christopher Reeve is who I have in mind, but Henry Cavill fits the bill just as well.) As long as I keep my intake of this trio adequate (along with collagen, without doubt the biggest contributor to the dermal upgrade), skin problems are a thing of the past. Their absence was my skin's kryptonite; and that was only the benefit I could *see*. Surely it did much more good on the inside.

If you struggle to find a good (and affordable) source of ghee, other natural sources of vitamin K2 are certain cheeses, natto (fermented soy, traditional Japanese food), beef and goose liver, the dark meat of chicken, and to some extent egg yolks. Or, simply supplement with K2 in capsule or pill form. The real thing is of course preferable to a pill, but sometimes you have to compromise. If I don't have any ghee at home, I simply get my Vitamin K2 in capsule form. Unless ghee is on sale (during which I stock up), it's pretty damn expensive here...

Supplements

I've cleaned up my supplement routine considerably; no more chlorella, goji berries or other so-called superfoods. They're expensive, often outrageously so, and in relation to their price, not worth it. You're better off eating regular (super) foods found at the supermarket, like turmeric, blueberries, salmon, sweet potatoes[34], onions, garlic, ginger[35], and liver[36].

The three things I do supplement my diet with are vitamin D, omega 3, and collagen. I don't do it religiously; if I've been out in the sun or had fish for dinner, I don't consume their capsule or pill equivalent. Collagen on the other hand is harder to come by, so I tend to supplement with it on a more regular basis. I've taken fish (or marine) collagen in the past, but now I take organic, grass-fed bovine collagen, in large part because it's cheaper here. Although our bodies make collagen, it is not enough for optimal health, and getting enough of it can promote youthful skin, improve joint health, improve digestion and reduce inflammation, and also improve wound healing.[37]

I noticed a difference in the appearance of my skin within a few weeks of starting to supplement with collagen; the enormous pores on my face got a lot smaller, the hue got somehow warmer, richer, and it felt less brittle (however out there that sounds).

Goodbye to the usual corpse-like tone and feel.

I want to really hammer this in: listen to your own body—personalization is key when it comes to food. What works for others might not work for you, and vice versa.

Look at your recent ancestry and what they ate[38], if any significant biological adaptations have been made[39], and at your own current circumstances.

Though diet is a huge contributor to my progress, I also have to credit other lifestyle-specific changes that I've incorporated into my routine; such as subjecting myself to extreme temperatures and doing breathing exercises, both courtesy of an amazing man named Wim Hof...

Courage is resistance to fear, mastery of
fear—not absence of fear.

Mark Twain

The Tragedy of Pudd'nhead Wilson and
the Comedy Those Extraordinary Twins
(1894)

Chest Freezers and Oxygen Junkies

A cold shower. The words alone would curl the hair at the back of my neck a few years ago. How about a cold bath then?

What? How is that better? No. Never!

Fast forward to today, and I actually look forward to my next cold session.

Yes... this will be uncomfortable. In the beginning. But take it easy; work your way down steadily. Nice and slow. Or, jump right in. However you choose to do it; be careful—it might soon turn into an addiction. Sooner than you think.

I thought it could never occur, my longing for a cold shower, but I actually do just that nowadays. And it's not just that I know that they do me good; there's something else at play here as well. It's almost like stepping into a different reality of sorts. Time doesn't stop; it dissolves. (Brace yourself for more woo-woo in the following passage.)

There's a point when you're submerged in the cold, enveloped by it, when you pass a threshold of sorts, a very physical sensation, when the cold becomes in some strange way comfortable. It's almost like a pleasant pseudo-shiver, scurrying around inside you, around your organs, on the inside of your skin, insulating you, solidifying you. Not only that, it calms me down, roots me; like a big blanket is lowered, lowered onto the soul, whispering sweet nothings to it. My breath slows down. My mind calms down. It's a very strange sensation, one I've never experienced outside of cold showers and baths. For lack of a better term, it's Zen.

Who knew you could find it in a freezer.

The many benefits the cold brings to your psyche are phenomenal; not only am I calmer, I've become more mentally resilient, and physically as well, in that I'm not as uncomfortable when I'm out in the cold anymore. Granted, these results are all subjective, but there's a plethora of anecdotal evidence out there praising the many benefits of cold showers and baths, as well as numerous studies that have been done. Hydrotherapy (in this case cold showers), can be a potential treatment for depression, increase circulation, strengthen your immune system[40], boost your mood, and increase alertness[41].

I'm only doing one side of the temperature equation, namely cold. But saunas have some great health benefits as well; they can improve athletic performance, lipid profiles, depression[42], potentially have some very interesting brain benefits like the growth of new brain cells, and also aid in detoxification[43].

I'm already seeing great results from just the cold; if I started doing some serious sauna time as well, I'd be unstoppable!

Let's hope. Right now I have about an hour's worth of sauna time in the last ten years. Not very impressive statistics…

That covers the first part of the Wim Hof Method—cold showers—the second being a breathing exercise. (There's actually a third one as well: commitment[44]. How else are you supposed to see any results?)

At first I did this sitting down, in what is called the Burmese position, or Sukhasana for those familiar with Yoga poses. (I wasn't familiar with either one until I looked up meditation and breathing positions for dummies.) But after a while I noticed that it feels better lying down. So I now do it lying flat on my back—the corpse position.

The exercise itself is very simple[45]:

- Take 30 deep breaths

- On the last exhalation, after you breathe out, emptying your lungs, simply hold it. Hold it until you feel the need to breathe again (but not so long that you feel like your eyes are going to explode)

- When you do breathe again, inhale once, deeply, and then hold it again; but this time for about 15 seconds

That's it. I usually do three rounds of this, a slight modification of the original routine. I do it pretty slow—slow and deep—and the first round of inhalations through my nose, the second round I do 15 through my nose and the next 15 through my mouth, and the third round I inhale through my mouth.

The very first couple of weeks I only did one round of 30 inhalations, marveling at how easy it was to do, but also how I never felt any of the effects that other people reported. Then I read it more carefully, and realized I had skipped quite a bit of it.

After the completed three rounds I experience a

sort of tingling sensation—often lighter sensations even after the first round—especially in my arms and legs, sometimes in my face as well, and also a pressure of sorts in the same areas. This is all perfectly normal. Once the three rounds are done, I feel like a million bucks; energized, revitalized, and overall pleasantly upbeat, in part from doing something beneficial (not only what I *believe* to be beneficial, though that probably plays a part as well).

I often put on some music before starting the breathing session; it's great to just lie there after it's done—as well as during the round intervals—listening to a good tune. It's meditation. Sometimes I skip the music and just breathe calmly in the silence instead.

What works best for me is to find a good rhythm, much slower than many of the instructional videos show, but still making sure that my body is getting saturated with oxygen. If I do it too fast my heart starts racing, and it doesn't even feel beneficial anymore, relaxing; just another inane stressor. If I do the opposite, do it too sloppily, my mind often starts to wander, and it feels completely wasted. Try to find a balance that works for you.

But be careful not to overdo it; I did it every day for a while, and soon found myself cutting corners wherever I could, just to get it over with. 25 inhales the first round, 23 on the second, and 20 on the last.

Or I'd do one giant mash-up, and do 50 inhalations at once; maybe 30 good ones and 20 sloppy ones. It had become a chore; something I'd much rather weasel out of. And weasel I did. So now I usually do the breathing exercises two to four times a week, and the cold showers two to four times a week as well, sometimes both on the same day, sometimes apart, sometimes right after each other, sometimes not. Sometimes less, sometimes more; it all depends on how I feel. (That was a lot of sometimes.) This way I don't weasel out of it, but actually enjoy doing it. After a while you get a sense of when it's appropriate to do them and when it's not, for instance, if I haven't slept well, then I don't take a cold shower, but I might do a breathing session. Listen to your body.

There's some very interesting science on the combination of cold exposure and the breathing exercise above: it can have beneficial effects on inflammation, pain, and stress resilience[46], as well as autoimmune conditions and psychiatric disorders[47]. Other possible benefits include better sleep, migraine relief, increased sports performance, faster recovery after exercise, more energy, asthma relief, lower blood pressure, and arthritis relief.[48]

Even though my immune system was already strengthened by the things I changed prior to implementing cold exposure and the breathing exercise, and even though I have only anecdotal evidence to present, I never get sick now. I mean that literally. I don't even remember the last time I had a cold. Even when spending time around the worst booger monsters of all; little children that just started kindergarten, rife with all kinds of fun invisible things to bring back home, and everyone else around me getting sick, I'm fine.

I have been assured by a very knowing
American of my acquaintance in London,
that a young healthy child well nursed is at
a year old a most delicious, nourishing,
and wholesome food, whether stewed,
roasted, baked, or boiled; and I make no
doubt that it will equally serve in a
fricassee or a ragout.

Jonathan Swift

A Modest Proposal For preventing the
Children of Poor People From being a
Burthen to Their Parents or Country, and
For making them Beneficial to the Publick
(1729)

How to Self-Eat (Cannibalize Yourself)

This might sound barbaric, and were you to chew on your arm, it might be. But nothing like that will be necessary. The basic idea of fasting is just to give your body ample time to process what you give it, and not to shove stuff in during every waking hour, keeping your digestive process on overdrive.

This is from Dr. Rhonda Patrick's website: "Fasting activates many of the body's mechanisms that repair damaged DNA and other cellular components. It also promotes the production of ketones, especially beta-hydroxybutyrate, an anti-aging molecule that demonstrates the capacity to delay the onset of aging-related diseases and improve mitochondrial health. There are several types of fasting, including alternate-day fasting, time-restricted eating, and prolonged fasting. Each elicits metabolic changes that can improve health and promote longevity. Time-restricted eating, in particular, has the potential to realign the body's circadian rhythms."[49]

I aim for a daily 8-hour window during which I eat, and the rest of it is spent fasting. Since I generally eat two meals a day, it's usually even less than that, say within a 6-hour window. Of course, sometimes it gets even shorter—like during days without workouts or much of any exertion, when I might only eat once a day—or sometimes that window is stretched in the other direction by a couple of hours. And sometimes it just doesn't work out at all. But that's the plan, anyway. For every day of the week.

I don't do 24-hour fasts anymore, or anything above 24 hours for that matter. For me, when fasting for longer than 24 hours, I feel strange. Strange in a bad way.

It turns out that fasting too long with fungal infections might not be a good idea.[50] So for me a too long fast means over 24 hours. It all depends on how it makes you feel.

The results aren't in on what exactly breaks a fast, but just to be on the safe side, I only consume water during the fasting periods—not even tea or coffee— just plain aqua, of the straight-from-the-tap kind.[51]

The benefits of fasting can include lower levels of inflammation[52], that you burn fat instead of sugar for energy (which leads to weight loss, as well as an improved cardiovascular disease risk profile), lower insulin and improved insulin sensitivity, increased levels of human growth hormone, increase your cells' resiliency and health, and improve your circadian rhythm[53].

Autophagy (from the Ancient Greek autóphagos, meaning self-devouring) "is the natural, regulated mechanism of the cell that removes unnecessary or dysfunctional components. It allows the orderly degradation and recycling of cellular components."[54] Other ways to induce autophagy besides fasting includes exercise[55], and possibly eating turmeric, drinking coffee and consuming olive oil as well[56].

If you're looking to detox, autophagy is the bona-fide way to go about it, the real way to cleanse your body.[57]

Most of the detox products people are pushing, like juices and powders, are pretty much useless. Our bodies have several built-in, natural and most importantly free means of getting rid of toxins, and these are excreted by breathing, urinating, defecating, and to some extent by sweating as well.

The first rule of Fight Cl—uh, I mean detox: don't put toxic stuff into your body.

But the walking of which I speak has nothing in it akin to taking exercise, as it is called, as the sick take medicine at stated hours—as the swinging of dumb-bells or chairs; but is itself the enterprise and adventure of the day. If you would get exercise, go in search of the springs of life. Think of a man's swinging dumb-bells for his health, when those springs are bubbling up in far-off pastures unsought by him!

Henry David Thoreau

June 1862 issue of The Atlantic Monthly

Keep Moving

Strongman competitions and triathlons for everyone! Or just go old-school Thoreau and swing some chairs while you go for a stroll through the neighborhood. Guaranteed to be therapeutic... or at the very least interesting.

I know this is getting tedious, but find what works for you. Strongman competitions and triathlons are far from everyone's cup of tea. Neither are structured forms of exercise. Find something that is easily incorporated into your daily life, isn't tedious or a downright punishment, and can be enjoyed many, many years from now.

Do as the Okinawans and other Blue Zoners do: dance, do Tai Chi, take long walks, run, swim, ride a bike; in short, put your muscles to use.[58] Also, sit less and move more throughout the day; even a seemingly trifle thing like getting up to walk around the office counts.[59]

"Blue Zones are regions of the world where Dan Buettner claims people live much longer than average. The term first appeared in his November 2005 National Geographic magazine cover story,

"The Secrets of a Long Life." Buettner identified five regions as "Blue Zones" (a term he trademarked): Okinawa (Japan); Sardinia (Italy); Nicoya (Costa Rica); Icaria (Greece); and among the Seventh-day Adventists in Loma Linda, California."[60]

There is also evidence that occasionally lifting heavy things and sprinting has its own benefits, as does high-intensity exercise: merging them (high-intensity strength training) might be even better.[61]

There's also ample evidence that exercise is beneficial against depression.[62]

Whatever you decide to do (an exercise smorgasbord, perhaps?), the important thing is to find something sustainable. Which is easier said than done...

There is also the danger of wanting to do too much at once when it comes to exercise; especially after discovering it may hold great benefits to your particular situation, risking not only disillusionment down the line but possible injuries befalling you as well in pursuit of health.

The perils of overtraining are several—for instance, it can have harmful effects on the immune system—so to reduce the risk of overtraining but still enjoy high-intensity workouts, Chris Kresser suggests the following: reduce the frequency, get adequate rest, mix it up, and make sure you get adequate amounts of carbohydrates.[63]

But don't be fooled thinking an hour or two of exercise over the weekend will make up for the past five days spent sitting. "A sedentary lifestyle, comprising prolonged sitting and minimal physical activity, has a negative effect on nearly every aspect of human health." And also this: "Some research even suggests that people who exercise intensely, like marathon runners, are more likely to be sedentary when they're not exercising, falsely assuming their training offers them the full benefits of exercise and protects them from the harmful effects of sitting. What's more, in some cases marathons, triathlons, and long-distance bicycle rides can result in overtraining, and studies have linked these activities with heart, muscle, and joint damage."[64]

My own exercise routine is centered on workouts at home and at the outdoor gym. Often that entails regular strength training or high-intensity strength training, as well as sprints. During summertime I also swim.

Sometimes I work out in a fasted state (toward the end of it) and then eat, thus breaking the fast, or I work out between meals, and occasionally I don't eat anything at all after a workout, unless it's a heavy session, and my whole body screams for some food. This is an effort to mimic our ancestors, whose eating patterns varied greatly—between times of plenty, and times of scarcity. Not every hunt was successful, nor was there always something to nibble on. Experiment with what feels good for you on a day to day basis—don't just go after what you've always been told. Become a gut whisperer.

I do deep bodyweight squats almost every day, 30 of them, either all at once or spread out over the course of the day, and maybe four or five times a week I do bodyweight pushups, also 30 repetitions, and a bodyweight back exercise called Angels and Devils[65]. This is on top of the training I do during the week. Sometimes I do calf raises instead, lunges, bodyweight Romanian deadlifts, some shadow boxing, or whatever pops into my head. Sometimes I find a new exercise that I want to try, so I do that instead.

I also switched to doing a deep bodyweight squat (sometimes called Asian squat or Slav squat) instead of bending over, which can retain athletic functioning, hip function, and mobility for life (the squat, not my reluctance to bend over).[66] Before every workout, I also do knee circles.[67] It's a good way to incorporate things you want to do on a more or less daily basis. Just make it a part of the warmup, and that way you'll never skip it. Before every workout I also do stability training; my brother got me a stability cushion (a plate-sized plastic pillow with little studs, half-inflated) on which I stand with one foot at a time, working on my balance. It adds up to less than five minutes a day in total, but I feel like it has made my balance a great deal better, something that many of my flare-ups in the past messed *with*, and consequently messed *up*.

I don't stretch anymore, either before or after a workout; in fact, I hardly stretch at all. Only when my calves are really sore, or something similar. When I feel like doing it, I do it, but not as part of a strict routine. There is no clear evidence that short static stretching (about 30 seconds) is of any benefit, whereas static stretching over 60 seconds might even be harmful; dynamic stretching (leg swings etc.) on the other hand, seem to be beneficial prior to workouts.[68]

When it comes to workout gear, I try to keep it as simple as possible. No fancy (or sexy) glow-in-the-dark leotards or fitness watches. No synthetic clothes, especially not the layer that's in contact with my skin; I opt for cotton clothes in the summer and merino wool during wintertime, both preferably organic. Because the amount of harmful chemicals in common workout clothing is worrying.[69]

Another thing that has had a big impact, on many levels, is working on my posture. "Poor posture is incredibly damaging, both to the individual and to society at large. The very obvious downside to poor posture is the debilitating physical pain that accompanies it. If you spend your days sitting, standing, and walking with a fundamentally flawed posture, you are going to be hurting. It may not hit you right away, but it will catch up with you, and if you want to live a long, active life a healthy back is pretty much required. Remember, too, that the spinal cord is essentially a high-bandwidth system for the transfer of information between nerves, organs, and other parts of our anatomy. If your posture is poor and your spine is impacted, some experts even suggest your ability to process information and relay data will be compromised."[70] Not only does improving your posture open up the ribcage, allowing you to breathe better, but it makes you feel solid too; not like a sack of old potatoes shuffling about. Jeff Cavaliere has a great video on posture and how to fix it.[71]

Incorporating it into your daily life might take a while, it certainly did for me, but the more I was conscious of it, the more I was conscious of my piss-poor posture, and the more I corrected it. I can't claim I have a proper posture at all times, but it's certainly much better. Be aware (beware!) that once you start correcting your own posture, you start to see the atrocious postures of other people. And a lot of people have downright appalling postures: some look like geese, some are S-shaped, and the more extreme cases are Z-shaped. Once you see them—the vulture necks, the prying guts—you can't unsee them.

And I can't take my eyes off them either; I've caught myself staring at people like they were upright zebras taking the subway.

I've started to walk barefoot a lot as well; unless I'm going out, I don't put any shoes on when I'm home. Not even slippers; only during wintertime do I put socks on. I've even bought myself minimalist or barefoot shoes; shoes that have a flat, thinner sole. The toe box is also considerably more spacious—no more sardine-can existence for my battered toes. This change forced me to become conscious of my gait, and it slowed me down too. I don't know why I hurried so much everywhere... (Or do I?)

Here's what Mark Sisson has to say about conventional shoes: "They sever our physical connection to the earth, perturb our natural running and walking gait, and probably increase our risk of running injuries by increasing the forces acting on our joints when we land." Further down on the same page: "I decided to write this because I've been to the other side and back. I spent a decade running hundreds of miles every week. As an endurance athlete, my choice of shoes was predicated on its ability to absorb the impact of the road and deaden my nerves enough to allow me to continue running hundreds of miles every week. But, after years of chronic injuries, poor posture, and tissue inflammation, I realized my errors and changed my ways. I've now spent the better part of a decade leading a barefoot-dominant lifestyle."[72]

I haven't worked out in an indoor gym for almost a decade now. At home I can blast whatever music I want, and there's no waiting involved or covert rubbernecking. It's not appealing anymore: outdoor gyms are so much nicer, and if they're close to—or *in* the forest—even better. For me exercising out in the open has so many things going for it compared to a stuffy, boring gym. The economical aspect being a huge one.

If there's no outdoor gym around, you can just work out in the forest, or a park, which hopefully has trees (unless you plan to do a ground-based workout). A rope is oftentimes all the equipment you need when there are trees around. Or simply an exploratory nature—if the monkey in you is alive and well.

I can get by on bodyweight exercises alone; some weeks I do just that, when I need a little break from the heavier, weight-focused workouts. I have a barbell and a few weights, as well as rubber bands at home. My brother also bought me parallettes (about knee-height) as well as rings that can be attached to pull-up bars or branches, which are great additions to my workout regimen. It keeps things fun and interesting.

Initially I started working out in an attempt to

level the playing field, or even to gain an upper hand
on a diseased body that failed to do as I wished. A
fuck you to a body that didn't listen to commands.
Bad dog... sit! Vanity played a big part too; I
imagined I could offset the cosmetic discrepancy
brought on by acne by building muscle. Maybe
people would disregard the horror on my chest, back,
butt (I wish), and face that way. If I was fierce.

But over time it became so much more. It was a
way to learn about the functions of the human body,
the movement patterns, the muscles, tendons, and
bones. And I often felt better *after* a workout, even if
I went in fatigued or had a severe case of the blues.
It's almost like meditation, a state of trance; whether
you're surrounded by great music, or the sound of the
wind rustling the leaves above you, everything else
but the exercise ahead and your breathing
disappears. For me, it's a great cerebral cleanser; a
cerebral flush of the best kind.

Of course, I also want to look good naked.[73]

It's also a type of insurance, both against injury
and illness. But working out can quickly become
more of a crutch than an aid; in the past, fear of
missing a single workout has kept me from enjoying
other, non-workout-related stuff. I measured myself
by the latest workout, and if I skipped a day, I felt like
a slob. I was restless too; I could be working out now
instead! Doing something beneficial!

As mentioned earlier, the weakness in the left side of my body has virtually disappeared. The strength imbalance I obsessed over for so long is at a point that I don't register a difference anymore.

Was it a vision, or a waking dream?
Fled is that music: — Do I wake or sleep?

John Keats

Ode to a Nightingale, Stanza 8 (1819)

Make Peace with the Sandman

The Sandman and I weren't on the best of terms back in the day. I frequently slept bad, had bouts of insomnia, and often woke up feeling so tired that it was as if the night had provided me no relief at all.

That's all changed now, thanks to the methods I put forth in the Feed thy Gut series. Sure, I occasionally have a bad night, as we all do. Especially when I go beyond my regular hours. But on the whole, I now sleep soundly.

Some time ago, I decided to try and simply go to bed whenever I felt tired in the evening. I decided to give it a week, and see what became of it. Within a few days I established that 21:00 was my perfect bed time. I woke up at 05:00 more or less every time and felt great. And I've continued with that ever since: to bed around 21:00, and then I wake up by myself at 05:00 or at the latest at 05:30. I don't even need to set the alarm.

I also threw out my old bed, which had begun sagging to the point that it felt like being in a hammock, and replaced it with a thin, one-inch mattress placed straight onto the floor.

Cold showers have a very peculiar thing about them; if I take one in the morning, it energizes me like few things could, but if I take one in the evening, I sleep like a baby. That is, if I don't take it five minutes before going to bed. About an hour before bedtime seems to be the minimum.

Now to the importance of sleep.

Sleep plays a vital role in maintaining optimal mental and physical health throughout life, it preps the brain for information input, facilitates information storage and the brain's self-cleaning mechanism: the glymphatic system, and provides a mechanism for information transfer and the formation of long-term memories, and a lack of sleep can impair glucose regulation and promote an obesogenic profile.[74]

Sleep is essential for basic maintenance and repair of the neurological, endocrine, immune, musculoskeletal and digestive systems. Sleep deprivation can lead to an impaired immune system, cognitive decline, systemic inflammation, and reduced lifespan. "And here's the thing: you can eat a perfect diet and take all the right supplements, but if you're not sleeping well and managing your stress, all bets are off."[75]

Ben Greenfield offers some valuable tips on getting a good night's sleep: fix your circadian rhythm, focus on good air quality (especially in the bedroom), optimize your body temperature, beware of sleep-disturbing substances, and time exercise properly.[76]

This was a short chapter, but making it into a chapter highlights the importance of sleep and establishing a good snooze routine. Onward!

Lecturer, n. One with his hand in your pocket, his tongue in your ear and his faith in your patience.

Clairvoyant, n. A person, commonly a woman, who has the power of seeing that which is invisible to her patron, namely, that he is a blockhead.

Admiration, n. Our polite recognition of another's resemblance to ourselves.

Circus, n. A place where horses, ponies and elephants are permitted to see men, women and children acting the fool.

Ambrose Bierce

The Devil's Dictionary (1911)

Everyday Tweaks

Let's follow the above list of quotes with a motley catalogue of adjustments I've made over the years:

The Body

- Squat poop (i.e. either have a stool under my feet to elevate them, or simply raise my heels as high off the floor as possible).

- No commercial toothpaste; I brush my teeth with baking soda, and sometimes with turmeric as well.

- No commercial shampoo. I rarely shampoo my hair, but if I do, I use either apple cider vinegar (ACV) or baking soda.

- The only stuff I put on my face is organic shea butter. Works great as both moisturizer and after shave.

- No perfumes. The ubiquitous scenting of products is a real health hazard.[77]

- No commercial deodorants. If I need some pit relief, I either use sea salt, baking soda, or apple cider vinegar.

- Microscopic plastic fibers cause a lot of harm on both land[78] and sea[79], and in all likelihood our foods are now full of them (as are we). Though the impact these plastics have on humans is not yet fully clear[80], I'm guessing it's not going to be in any way beneficial. So synthetic clothing is verboten on the Christmas wish list. Santa will come knocking in a makeshift hemp-sack poncho.

At Home

- No commercial dishwashing liquid. If needed, I use ACV. As for hand soap, I rarely have a use for it; water gets rid of most grime, and what's left (unless I dropped something in a cesspit) I can live with. Again, ACV comes in handy here too.

- No commercial cleaners: ACV alone is often

enough, but ACV combined with baking soda gets rid of even the nastiest of filth. If you want it scented, just put some lemon juice in it.

- No commercial washing detergents. I use baking soda (sodium bicarbonate) in a pinch, but soda ash (sodium carbonate) is the optimal pick.

- Use houseplants that are good air cleaners.[81]

Our business in this world is not to succeed, but to continue to fail, in good spirits.

Robert Louis Stevenson

Reflections and Remarks on Human Life (1878)

The Brain Game

Over the last couple of years, I've focused more and more on something I pretty much neglected before: my mental diet. Sure, that became much easier once I got a better grasp on the food part, once it was smoothly integrated into my daily life and I could do it blindfolded, so to speak. But the food part would've probably gone a lot smoother had I broadened my scope a bit. *Probably*. Or maybe not.

First order of business was to get rid of the distractions. The kangaroo in the rabbit pen was social media; internet as a whole. Of course, it can be a marvelous asset, a way into a whole new world; but that's not the primary way in which I went about it. The amount of time I wasted on the internet…

I never was much into social media to begin with (being a loner), which is probably why it was so easy to give it up completely. I do have an old smartphone, but I made it deliberately dumb; there's no internet on it, so its only functions are calls, texts, and taking pictures. The peace of mind from having a dumbphone, the bodily harmony it brings, is mindboggling.

Of course, I still sometimes waste my time online, but less rarely, and I'm able to stop it fairly early since a nagging voice materializes, drowning everything else out. I'm much more selective about how I spend my time online now; what I do, what I watch or listen to, what I read.

An odd consequence of this was that it made me think, obsessively for a time, about ideals, and my role in it. I realized I had boxed myself in; constructed an ideal I can't possibly live up to. I can't deviate from my diet even one bit. I can't feel sad anymore either... heaven forbid I become depressed again! I can't lie to people. I have a responsibility now!

Oh, the delusions...

Because I'm so famous, and so virtuous: Dalai "Drama" Lama!

It might be that I'm unusually obstinate, or just merely on this issue, but I'm not quitting this any time soon. Sure, there'll be ups and downs along the way, that's a given. But one of the best feelings I've ever had was when I realized that this is all actually working; the countless hours spent reading up on things, experimenting, abstaining, failing—it all paid off. Of course, I would've preferred a straighter trajectory, a faster one, but that would've surely presented problems of its own. In this case, slow and steady wins the race.

And it's not like I'm chasing some kind of lost high again; if you're going after something which to you is a legitimate goal, and you're making real progress, you're going to keep pursuing it. It gives life meaning.

I can be deep too.

Whether you stick to it 95, 85, or 75 percent of the time doesn't matter. Whatever number it takes to stick to it, to keep on pushing through, you take it.

But there is however a certain threshold that needs to be reached to see any sort of benefits; you can't do 25 percent and expect something great to happen. But 100 percent might be equally bad, if you're constantly trying to find shortcuts or ways to wriggle out of the shackles. That's when I start to sabotage things for myself.

It's better to start too low and up it later than to come out blasting and then fall back to where you started (or worse), never to try again. To stay on course you need a bit of iniquity. Yin and Yang motherfucker!

Sorry, that was uncalled for. My deepest apologies.

And it doesn't have to be for all eternity; you have to see how you feel, how your body responds, how it heals; you alone decide how far you want to take it, how long each phase lasts, or how long you're willing to keep it up for.

If you want to go back to a diet of pizzas and burgers, that's your choice too. But why eat crap?

Once you've been to the other side, or even just peeked over the fence, seen what difference it can make to your life, why go back?

But I guess it just makes it all the more easier to fall, once you begin to climb the metaphorical rungs of the ladder. And this is scary. Because you can't do more than try your best. There's always an element of the uncertain lurking about. The dark hole is, in a way, safety.

And being sick is itself a comfort of sorts; it's one of the best excuses, if not the best. An excuse to yourself and to those around you. To procrastinate, to avoid. To avoid harm.

The control freak in me is alive and well. One that at times thought it better to orchestrate my own demise rather than to let go and simply watch; and other times it presented a handy scapegoat: of course this approach didn't work out—good—now I can go back to the old ways of going about things. To safety.

The Devil you know is better than the one you don't. Or so the saying goes, anyway...

(So, by extension, I'm the Devil? That's not news, nor is it anything to pat myself on the head for. Every creature in every pantheon resides within every human's psyche. At least I sincerely hope so. Life would be very boring if that wasn't the case.)

Nowadays, when I'm about to sabotage myself in the food department, I take a step back—mentally as

well as physically at times—to really drive it home:
wait. Think about this. Think of what you're about to
do.

I can't say I succeed every time, but it's getting
much better.

With other things too, like fasting and exercise.
I'm not as hard on myself as I used to be. If I skip a
workout, or go over the allotted hours; don't sweat it.
Try again the next day. Same goes for whether or not
you'll be able to abide by the "don't sweat it" line.

Do I still think of myself as someone with MS?
Someone that *suffers* from MS?

Suffers? Hmm. I want to say never, but that's not
true. It happens. But very rarely. During moments
when I feel particularly sorry for myself. But as
someone *with* MS? The label of MS will forever be
attached to my body, tattooed on it, no matter what
happens. But I don't think about MS, or even of
myself as having it very often. Sometimes when the
word pops up, whatever the circumstances, I go: oh
yeah, I have MS too! But at the same time as I feel a
sort of kinship... it's a poisoned sort of kinship. I
don't go to checkups anymore; no MRIs; no doctor or
neurologist has called; no one has expressed any
interest in me (or my methods). Last one was about
ten years ago, and that was to tell me that they don't
think quitting the medication was a smart move. I'm
in no-man's land now: I'm not part of the healthy

population, and I'm not welcome into the world of sick people either. Some days I love it, some days I don't.

(Maybe this dogged polarization of mine is part of the problem...)

That also begs the question; where the hell am I then?

I guess time will tell...

(Once I furnish the hole I dug out for myself. In the wall. Peeper!)

Since I'm doing this all on my own, basically trying my way forward, it's bound to take longer than if I went to a specialist. But back when I started all this, there were no specialists like that in Sweden. All the stuff I read about and the persons deep in it were abroad, mostly in the United States.

I've lost a great deal of faith in the medical establishment, particularly when it comes to treating chronic disease.

But I also enjoy doing all of this... I think. Or did I simply force myself into enjoying it out of necessity, so I could justify it, so I wouldn't go crazy?

In the end, am I in a better place than I was? Am I happier?

In response to the first question, definitely. As to the happiness part, is that even a legitimate aim? Aren't things like happiness best achieved as unintended side effects? Not as aims in themselves?

Aim for something worth your while. Something that makes you want to get up in the morning.

And if people tell you something is wrong, ask why. Why is it wrong? Who thinks it's wrong?

The thing you want to do the least is oftentimes the very thing you need to do the most; the thing that will be of most benefit to you. Which, again, is scary. But how can I expect to gain anything of value from something which I invest nothing of myself in? Something that has little meaning to me (or anyone else)?

It's nuanced. Oh, it sure is...

"Look at that blacksmith, for instance,"
went on Father Brown calmly; "a good
man, but not a Christian—hard,
imperious, unforgiving. Well, his Scotch
religion was made up by men who prayed
on hills and high crags, and learnt to look
down on the world more than to look up at
heaven. Humility is the mother of giants.
One sees great things from the valley; only
small things from the peak."

G. K. Chesterton

The Hammer of God, published in the
short story collection The Innocence of
Father Brown (1911)

Poser

I thought long and hard about whether to include a picture or two in addition to the text, some visual proof, like I did in the first book; but this time including something of a much more agreeable nature. And of course that involved me getting undressed. (Forgive me, Father... Brown, for I am about to pose sinfully.)

Because for the most part, pictures do speak louder than words. But how the hell am I going to do that? I never kept a video diary, or even the occasional photograph of my journey. (Except for the toenail horror featured in the first book. Astute choice.) What is an impactful image, other than the fact that I'm alive and breathing? (Supposedly.) Me doing a handstand? I can't even do a freestanding handstand. Grinning in front of the produce aisle?

How can I somehow "prove" all these claims I'm making?

By flexing! That's how...

And yes, it is a little naughty too. Perhaps. Or maybe my naughtiness gauge needs calibrating... shut up already and strike a pose!

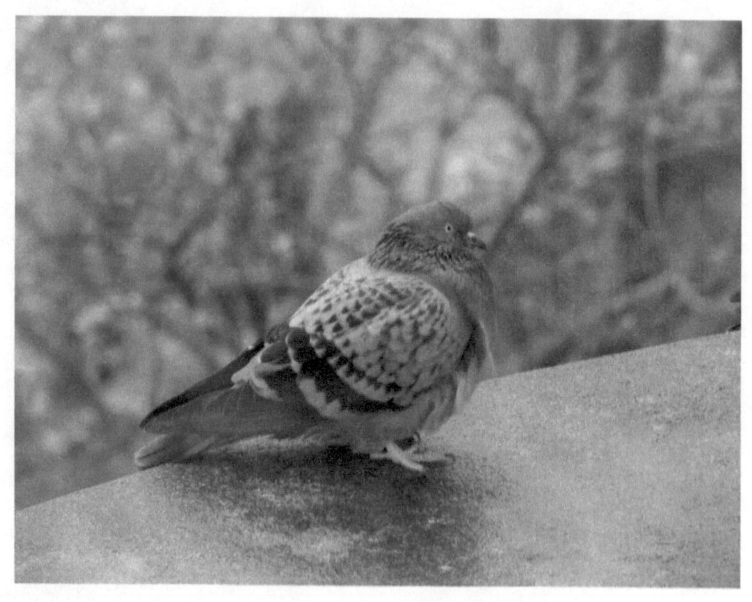

(Aww... come on!)

But is a muscular body proof of a *healthy* body?

To some extent. A very limited extent? Perhaps. Roid rage!

But feeling good about my own body is important to me. And exercising has definitely helped me with that, both in the aesthetic sense, and more importantly, the functional sense. The benefits have no doubt spilled over to other areas as well.

In a way, I took control of it, molded it to my own liking, strengthened it, instead of merely listening to the dire dictums of the well-meaning but ill-informed doctors.

Do I work out to be content with my body, or do I work out to feel better overall? Definitely the second part—the immense benefits of exercise are irrefutable—but it sure would be harder to do, to put in the work, without the visual feedback.

Which is vain, I guess, but then again I am vain. And occasionally extremely vain. No refutation necessary. Call me Mr. Vain...

(Dance pause!)

I have basically no weight fluctuations since adopting the methods put forth here and in the previous book, only when I gain muscle mass (nice humble brag), but other than that, I stay in great shape year round (again!).

At the end of the day, it is something I'm proud of; it required dedication, grit, and a bit of ingenuity. When I was eighteen I envisioned myself in a wheelchair in the span of a couple of years, or at least a cane (come on, give me something!). It might've never come to that at all—who knows where I'd be had I not taken this path—but the way things were progressing the first couple of years after the diagnosis... it did not bode well for the future.

From time to time, I still stand in my underwear in front of the bathroom mirror, flex, and then go: yeah, motherfucker, this is MS; sometimes I even say it out loud. (Good thing I'm close to the toilet, since that's

probably what my expression most resembles.)
I'll let your imagination play with that one.

Wickedness is a myth invented by good
people to account for the curious
attractiveness of others.

Oscar Wilde

Phrases and Philosophies for the Use of
the Young (1894)

The List

Welcome to the summary, also called *the just-fucking-tell-me-what-to-do list*.

The basic foundation to try and optimize: diet, sunshine exposure, sleep, exercise, relationships, and managing stress.

Add-ons: fasting, cold and/or heat exposure, walking barefoot, and doing meditation or breathing exercises.

My diet is as follows:

Carbohydrates

Potatoes
Sweet potatoes
White rice

Fruits

Berries
Bananas
Occasionally other fruits too

Vegetables and root vegetables

All of them!
(Including garlic, in all its forms, and also ginger—a
true superstar when it comes to health benefits[82].)

Fats

Ghee (good source of vitamin K2 in the ADK trio)
Extra virgin olive oil
Coconut oil (but only rarely)
Avocados

Meat

All meats, organ meats, fish, and seafood.
(As to organ meats, it's mostly liver. A great source of
vitamin A in the ADK trio.)

Supplements

Vitamin D (do I need to add that it's a vital part of the ADK trio?)
Omega 3
Collagen

Other foods

Eggs (optimal is three a day, as recommended by The Perfect Health Diet)
Cacao/Cocoa beans
Seeds (pumpkin, sunflower, sesame, flax, poppy—most of the time I eat them lightly roasted)
Spices: turmeric, black pepper, white pepper, cayenne pepper and other chili peppers, cinnamon, cumin, caraway, fennel seeds, nutmeg, mustard seeds, cloves, saffron, thyme, oregano, rosemary, nettles, peppermint... the list can be made very long. But do include some of them at least, since they contain very valuable compounds.[83] (Instead of chewing bubblegum, try sucking on some cloves, fennel seeds, coriander seeds, cardamom seeds[84], or fresh mint leaves.)

I also buy sea salt with dried seaweed in it for the iodine.

Sometimes

Nuts. I eat between one to three Brazil nuts a week (for the selenium); almonds, walnuts, cashews, hazelnuts, and pistachios I eat less frequently, or hardly at all; and peanuts I steer clear of altogether.

A little sincerity is a dangerous thing, and
a great deal of it is absolutely fatal.

Oscar Wilde

The Critic as Artist, Part II (1891)

Thanksgiving: 2nd Edition

Wim Hof. This man and his methods changed my life for the better to an extent I couldn't even have imagined (especially considering the freezing part); he helped me to take bodily healing to another level altogether, not to mention the benefits the cold brought to my mental makeup. (I'm far from the only one to have benefitted from his methods. A quick online search will give you plenty to be inspired by.) If you haven't heard of this man and his methods, go look him up.

Paul Jaminet and Shou-Ching Shih Jaminet and their very informative (and for me game-changing) book "The Perfect Health Diet". Their website (perfecthealthdiet.com) is also loaded with useful information; the Q&A section on there is particularly helpful, where Paul Jaminet himself answers questions.

Jeff "Athlean X" Cavaliere, and his many excellent

training videos. He provides consistently high-quality content, very science oriented (I learned a great deal about the human body from him), and also which exercises are bad and which ones are much better alternatives. Simply put, he makes it very easy to train smart. And since I do my training either at home or at outdoor gyms, his extensive knowledge, as well as countless ingenious tips and tricks, are invaluable.

T-Nation.com (Testosterone Nation). Especially Christian Thibaudeau, Ben Bruno, Gareth Sapstead, Bret Contreras, Chad Waterbury, Nick Tumminello, and Tony Gentilcore. It sounds hardcore—Testosterone Nation—and I guess it is compared to many other training sites, but the level of expertise is astonishing, not to mention the boatloads of inspiration I've gathered from their many articles and videos.

As for the mental diet, there are few people that have nourished the walnut like Joe Rogan and his podcast The Joe Rogan Experience (JRE). Where to even begin with this one? The amount of knowledge on there is astounding, not to mention the entertainment value. And from virtually every field imaginable; that's the beauty of it, that it's so eclectic. This was also where I first heard of Dr. Rhonda

Patrick, who has since given me many health-related delicacies. Her own website and podcast, FoundMyFitness, is also chockfull of interesting and educating material. JRE also provide me with the luxury of listening in on conversations with other health-related people, like Chris Kresser, Mark Sisson, and Robb Wolf. Among many, many, many other interesting episodes.

JRE was also where I first encountered Eric Weinstein; a very original thinker with an astounding mind. Though some of the things he talks about fly over my head, the things I do pick up are more often than not equally brilliant and disturbing (in the best sense). His own podcast, The Portal, is a real gem.

Dr. Jordan B Peterson. I first came across him through the audio version of his first book, "Maps of Meaning: The Architecture of Belief". It was incredibly absorbing, so I decided to get his latest book as well, watching (rather aimlessly) random clips of his until it arrived, to get a sense of who he was. In a matter of days I had his new book "12 Rules for Life" in my hand; a book that improved my mental landscape in all its vastness for the better like few (if any) books have accomplished in the past. A truly transformational read. Of course, after that I wanted even more, and boy oh boy, does his channel come through. But this time I went about it differently. His eponymous YouTube channel is chockfull of educational videos; interviews, debates, and a whole lot of great lectures, most of them on psychology. I get a world-class education sitting halfway across the globe, and I can pause whenever I want, either to look something up or just to chew something over—I'm terribly spoiled that way. Even though I wasn't brought up with any particular sort of religion (unless you count staunch atheism), I found his Bible lectures[85] absolutely fascinating.

Never put off till to-morrow what you can
do day after to-morrow just as well.

Signed "B.F." but actually written by Mark
Twain

"The Galaxy" magazine (1870)

The Denouement

It's almost over now... In relation to the quote above, there is a longer passage about Benjamin Franklin (B.F.) at the very end of a piece Mark Twain wrote for The Galaxy magazine in their July 1870 issue[86], which puts the aforementioned quote in some context:

"Benjamin Franklin did a great many notable things for his country, and made her young name to be honored in many lands as the mother of such a son. It is not the idea of this memoir to ignore that or cover it up. No; the simple idea of it is to snub those pretentious maxims of his, which he worked up with a great show of originality out of truisms that had become wearisome platitudes as early as the dispersion from Babel; and also to snub his stove, and his military inspirations, his unseemly endeavor to make himself conspicuous when he entered Philadelphia, and his flying his kite and fooling away his time in all sorts of such ways, when he ought to have been foraging for soap-fat, or constructing

candles. I merely desired to do away with somewhat
of the prevalent calamitous idea among heads of
families that Franklin acquired his great genius by
working for nothing, studying by moonlight, and
getting up in the night instead of waiting till morning
like a Christian, and that this programme, rigidly
inflicted, will make a Franklin of every father's fool.
It is time these gentlemen were finding out that these
execrable eccentricities of instinct and conduct are
only the evidences of genius, not the creators of it. I
wish I had been the father of my parents long enough
to make them comprehend this truth, and thus
prepare them to let their son have an easier time of it.
When I was a child I had to boil soap,
notwithstanding my father was wealthy, and I had to
get up early and study geometry at breakfast, and
peddle my own poetry, and do every thing just as
Franklin did, in the solemn hope that I would be a
Franklin some day. And here I am."

I didn't know where else to put this—or that erectile
dysfunction was reimagined by an ad agency so that a
pharmaceutical company could sell drugs to healthy
people[87]—but felt that I had to include it all
somewhere, somehow. And so it became a fitting way
to wrap up the book... you thinking of Mark Twain's
impish ghost, and dick pills.

And with that I shall bid you farewell. Godspeed.

See you all in health!

References

1.

https://draxe.com/nutrition/7-raw-garlic-benefits-reversing-disease/

2.

https://olivewellnessinstitute.org/article/garlic-in-low-fodmap/

3.

https://www.sciencedirect.com/science/article/abs/pii/S1756464614001376

4.

https://alittlebityummy.com/is-fermented-cabbage-sauerkraut-actually-low-fodmap/

5.

https://www.livescience.com/16556-spicy-food-fatal-chili-peppers.html

6.

https://draxe.com/nutrition/fructans-fructan-intolerance/

Here is a very interesting breakdown of "Dietary fructose intolerance, fructan intolerance and FODMAPs":
https://www.ncbi.nlm.nih.gov/pmc/articles/PMC3934501/

7.
https://www.healthline.com/nutrition/11-reasons-to-eat-berries

8.
https://www.amymyersmd.com/2018/03/keto-diet-autoimmune-disease/

9.
https://selfhack.com/blog/dr-paul-jaminet-the-ideal-diet-combatting-infections-gut-health-and-circadian-rhythms/

10.
https://chriskresser.com/episode-15-dr-paul-jaminet-on-chronic-infections-depression-more/

11.
https://en.wikipedia.org/wiki/Gut-brain_axis

12.
https://chriskresser.com/the-gut-skin-connection-how-altered-gut-function-affects-the-skin/

13.
https://en.wikipedia.org/wiki/Hygiene_hypothesis

14.
https://www.livescience.com/52344-inflammation.html

15.
https://chriskresser.com/why-you-should-think-twice-about-vegetarian-and-vegan-diets/

16.
https://chriskresser.com/the-carnivore-diet-is-it-really-healthy/

17.
https://chriskresser.com/red-meat-it-does-a-body-good/

18.
https://chriskresser.com/what-is-nutrient-density-and-why-is-it-important/

19.

https://podcastnotes.org/joe-rogan-experience/chris-kresser-joe-rogan-game-changers-vegan-diet/

20.
https://chriskresser.com/shifting-from-shock-awe-to-nourish-support/

21.
https://www.marksdailyapple.com/should-you-eat-less-protein/

22.
https://www.marksdailyapple.com/8-signs-you-probably-dont-need-more-protein/

23.
https://en.wikipedia.org/wiki/Ghee

24.
https://www.hindustantimes.com/health-and-fitness/soak-rice-overnight-to-reduce-risk-of-heart-diseases-cancer/story-6EoqUca3RfoqDouqo21xSP.html

25.
http://perfecthealthdiet.com/the-diet/

26.
https://www.westonaprice.org/proper-preparation-of-grains-and-legumes-video-by-sarah-pope/

27.
https://draxe.com/nutrition/ghee-benefits/

28.
https://www.westonaprice.org/health-topics/abcs-of-nutrition/on-the-trail-of-the-elusive-x-factor-a-sixty-two-year-old-mystery-finally-solved/

29.
https://chriskresser.com/vitamin-k2-the-missing-nutrient/

30.
https://draxe.com/nutrition/vitamin-k2/

31.
https://www.westonaprice.org/health-topics/know-your-fats/why-butter-is-better/

32.
https://paleoleap.com/preventing-and-healing-tooth-decay/

33.

https://www.drstevenlin.com/crooked-teeth-genetic/

Here is a great breakdown of Dr. Weston Price's findings regarding both dental health and health overall: https://www.westonaprice.org/health-topics/abcs-of-nutrition/the-right-price/

34. https://draxe.com/nutrition/what-are-superfoods/

35. https://www.marksdailyapple.com/6-hidden-superfoods-you-probably-already-have-in-your-pantry/

36. https://chriskresser.com/natures-most-potent-superfood/

37. https://www.maxlugavere.com/blog/why-you-should-add-more-collagen-to-your-diet

38. https://www.marksdailyapple.com/the-definitive-guide-to-using-your-recent-ancestry-to-determine-your-optimal-diet/

39.
https://www.nationalgeographic.com/culture/food/the-plate/2016/03/02/a-twist-on-paleo-eat-what-your-family-ate-500-years-ago/

40.
https://www.maxlugavere.com/blog/7-reasons-why-you-should-consider-taking-cold-showers

41.
https://www.medicalnewstoday.com/articles/325725#stronger-immune-system

42.
https://chriskresser.com/the-health-benefits-of-saunas/

43.
https://www.foundmyfitness.com/episodes/biohacker-summit-2016

44.
https://www.wimhofmethod.com/practice-the-method

45.
https://www.wimhofmethod.com/breathing-

exercises

46.
https://www.wimhofmethod.com/science

47.
https://www.sciencedaily.com/releases/2018/02/18
0228164934.htm

48.
https://www.wimhofmethod.com/benefits

For some very interesting videos on (and with) Wim
Hof, see these links:
https://www.foundmyfitness.com/episodes/pierre-
capel
https://www.foundmyfitness.com/episodes/wim-hof

49.
https://www.foundmyfitness.com/episodes/what-
type-of-fasting-is-best-rhonda-patrick

50.
http://perfecthealthdiet.com/q-a/comment-page-
29/
(See Paul Jaminet's comment on July 29, 2012 at
7:54 pm)
There's also more information in The Perfect Health

Diet book.

51.
https://www.foundmyfitness.com/episodes/satchin-round-2

52.
https://draxe.com/time-restricted-eating/

53.
https://chriskresser.com/intermittent-fasting-the-science-behind-the-trend/

54.
https://en.wikipedia.org/wiki/Autophagy

55.
https://www.foundmyfitness.com/topics/autophagy

56.
https://www.marksdailyapple.com/7-ways-to-induce-autophagy/

57.
https://www.ajc.com/lifestyles/health/autophagy-the-real-way-cleanse-your-body/o6qE9DQ4oT2hJ5hMNM1NpM/

58.
https://www.bluezones.com/2018/01/what-exercise-best-happy-healthy-life/

59.
https://www.bluezones.com/2020/01/the-neat-way-to-exercise-for-a-longer-healthier-life/

60.
https://en.wikipedia.org/wiki/Blue_Zone

61.
https://chriskresser.com/9-steps-to-perfect-health-7-move-like-your-ancestors/

62.
https://www.foundmyfitness.com/episodes/exercise-depression

63.
https://chriskresser.com/why-you-may-need-to-exercise-less/

64.
https://chriskresser.com/why-you-need-to-move-every-day-to-get-the-benefits-of-exercise/

65.

https://www.youtube.com/watch?v=FmeJeomoSN8
"7 "SISSY" Exercises for "BAD ASS" Muscle Gains!"
At 1:25 the Angels and Devils exercise starts. Doing it
without weights is more than sufficient.

66.
https://www.t-nation.com/training/tip-do-a-deep-
bodyweight-squat-daily

67.
https://www.youtube.com/watch?v=99mL_3Zk7BI
"Knee Strengthening Exercise to Keep Knees
Healthy"

68.
https://www.marksdailyapple.com/are-stretching-
and-warmups-overrated/

69.
https://www.shape.com/fitness/clothes/harmful-
chemicals-hidden-your-workout-clothes

70.
https://www.marksdailyapple.com/improve-
posture/

71.
https://www.youtube.com/watch?v=TQqgf8kB6R8

"Perfect Posture in 5 Steps (BAD POSTURE
BUSTER!)"

He has more videos on that topic, for instance this:
https://www.youtube.com/watch?v=g-7ZWPCWv0U
"How to Fix Your Posture in 4 Moves!
(PERMANENTLY)"

72.
https://www.marksdailyapple.com/how-to-safely-
and-enjoyably-transition-to-a-barefoot-dominant-
lifestyle/

73.
https://www.marksdailyapple.com/health-vanity/

74.
https://www.foundmyfitness.com/episodes/matthe
w-walker

75.
https://chriskresser.com/9-steps-to-perfect-health-
8-sleep-more-deeply/

76.
https://bengreenfieldfitness.com/article/sleep-
articles/increase-deep-sleep/

77.
https://www.theguardian.com/us-news/2019/may/23/fragrance-perfume-personal-cleaning-products-health-issues

78.
https://www.npr.org/sections/thesalt/2017/02/06/511843443/are-we-eating-our-fleece-jackets-microfibers-are-migrating-into-field-and-food?

79.
https://grist.org/living/2011-12-07-how-microplastics-cause-macro-problems-for-the-ocean/

80.
https://www.discovermagazine.com/health/microplastics-are-everywhere-but-their-health-effects-on-humans-are-still

81.
https://lifehacker.com/this-graphic-shows-the-best-air-cleaning-plants-accord-1705307836

82.
https://draxe.com/nutrition/10-medicinal-ginger-health-benefits/

83.

https://draxe.com/nutrition/top-herbs-spices-healing/

84.
https://draxe.com/nutrition/cardamom/

85.
https://www.youtube.com/watch?v=f-wWBGo6a2w
"Biblical Series I: Introduction to the Idea of God"

86.
The Mark Twain article in its entirety—which is marvelous—can be found here:
http://www.twainquotes.com/Galaxy/187007e.html

87.
https://www.ncbi.nlm.nih.gov/pmc/articles/PMC14 34483/